Zen and the Art of Illness

Ronna Fay Jevne

Praise for Zen & the Art of Illness

Dr. Jevne knows, through both personal and professional experience, about serious illness and poor prognosis. This eloquent book will touch your very core as you experience her being present in and surrendering to the moment, and of letting go of the need to "do" - the true essence of Zen. The story moves us to see that our real journey in life is interior and is made up of a series of firsts. You will be witness to how one keeps hope alive at the edge of death and how one can co-habit with uncertainty; transcending the probable and attending to the possible. This powerful book will leave you changed as you face life's challenges.
Kaye Herth, Dean Emeritus, Minnesota State University, Mankato

---

This is a great book - tender, insightful, highly educational. It is a wonderful testimony to the love of two people. It describes an amazing and courageous journey, one filled with so much sadness and worry, yet with so much hope.
Mike Bell. former cancer patient, Inukshuk Management Consultants

---

I soon came to the realization that I had been invited to share in a Gift of the Sacred. Ronna reminds us that despite our circumstances, we can find and define choices, for ourselves when seemingly there are no choices and our backs are up against a wall. She truly portrays what it means to partner through the illness experience. Together, she and Allen model how to partner with a health care system that was not always "cooperative or logical" in a respectful way. This book offers hope and a voice for those who are walking the path of suffering through the experience of illness. It invites people living the experience to live in the moment and it shows, by example, ways it can be done.
Sharon Moore, Professor, Centre for Nursing & Health Studies. Athabasca University

Praise for Zen & the Art of Illness

What stayed with me having read, *Zen and the Art of Illness* is the sense of steadiness in the swirl of life and death. The practice of Zen comes shining through, as both Allen and Ronna carry a stillness through intense emotion, intrusive medical intervention, and moments of inner and outer chaos. This is a very moving book.
<u>Kuya Minague</u>, *resident priest at Sakuraji, affiliate of the Silent Thunder Order*

Zen and the Art of Illness is a book that powerfully grips you as a reader and pulls you through the story to its end. The honesty about who they – Ronna and Allen – are, individually and as a couple, combined with the same honesty about their relationship with illness and this current illness journey leaves you both joyful and tearful, sometimes at the same moment. *Zen and the Art of Illness* shows us how everyday moments can be filled with meaning, conveying love, care, and respect. Conversely, it points out how the need for power and control, not listening, and ignoring what is said, can cause real harm. Indeed, we need to both understand and challenge the fact that: "It is the way of the system. It saves your life by taking it." (p. 45) Throughout the story, we are reminded of the value of presence as we negotiate illness journeys individually and together. A strong statement about life, illness, hope and meaning, *Zen and the Art of Illness* is a must-read.
<u>Christi Simpson,</u> *Phd., Head and Associate Professor, Department of Bioethics, Faculty of Medicine, Dalhousie University*

Other books by R. Jevne

- Living Life as a Writer
- Celebrating 60: Impulsive meditations on six decades.
- Tea for the Inner Me: Blending tea with reflection.
- Images and Echoes: (Editor) Exploring your life with photograpy and writing.
- Hoping coping and moping: Handling life when illness makes it tough.
- It all begins with hope: Patients, caregivers and the bereaved speak out.
- Voice of hope: Heard across the heart of life.
- Hope in practice: Selected conversations. (Editor)
- Louis' Path.

Co-authored

- Finding hope: Seeing the world in a brighterlight. With J. Miller
- No time for nonsense: Self help for the seriously ill. With A. Levitan
- Striving for health: Living with broken dreams. With H. Zingle
- When dreams don't work: Professional caregivers and burnout. With D. Williamson
- The Hope Journal: With J. Gurnett

Zen
and the
Art of Illness

Publisher: Prairie Wind Writing Centre
Millet, Alberta

Cover photo by Ronna Jevne

Copyright ©2017 Prairie Wind Writing Centre

All rights reserved. No part of this book may be reproduced in any form or by any means, electronic or mechanical, including photocopying, recording, or by any information storage or retrieval system, without permission in writing from the Prairie Wind Writing Centre except by a reviewer who may quote brief passages in review. First edition.

ISBN # 978-1-894045-07-0

Dedication

To Allen

You are my miracle

and

To:
Dr. Debra Jeffrey
Dr. Toni Reiman
Dr. Raeleen Cherry

Without whom hope and illness
could not have been
on an equal playing field.

Acknowledgments

The capacity to be in the moment is a lifetime practice. With time, I have come to understand that freedom comes with acknowledging reality, not with the effort to avoid it. A special thank you to Kuya Monague, for helping me deepen the practice of being here in this moment. Thank you Allen for never losing hope. Thank you family and friends for being there in the ways that you were able. Thank you to all who have walked this path before we walked it and for having compassion for those who have yet to visit the landscape of suffering and uncertainty. Thank you Hal, for your support in launching *Zen and the Art of Illness.*

Thanks to every person who works to sustain a health care system that recognizes that each of us is only a diagnosis away from being a victim of circumstances beyond our control. Because of you, we had access to treatment without threatening our future or limiting our choices.

We have an appointment with life, and that appoinntment takes place in the present moment.

> Thich Nhat Hahn

Table of Contents

Praise for *Zen and the Art of Illness*	2
Dedication and Acknowledgments	6
Introduction	10
PRE-DIAGNOSIS: Waiting in uncertainty	17
IN-PATIENT: Living in a medical culture	41
OUT-PATIENT: In limbo, but home	85
RETURNING TO LIFE: Finding normal again	133
Epilogue & Epilogue 2	164

Introduction

It was a time when life was supposed to get gentler, a time when there would be the resources for pampering a body and soul that had done 24/7 for 30 years. Time to play and host. Time to write and do photography and create. Time to be off the center of the stage. Time for freedom.

It was a time that turned on a dime. Turned to surrendering to reality, the reality that life and death were a possibility most days. Turned to mature sacrifice, without resentment. It was a time, not of fear, but of gratitude. Gratitude for the time we have stolen from fate. Time to live together with hope, despite the raging cancer.

It was a time of special moments, a time of memory making. A time of unspoken allegiance. A time when my appointment with life was today.

Journal Entry October, 2008

Zen and the Art of Illness

On February 12th 2008, my husband Allen was diagnosed with a high grade non-Hodgkin's lymphoma. In a matter of weeks, he went from a six-foot relatively vibrant 75 year old who had recently returned to university to take his third degree to a 129 pound frail elderly man. The cancer swept into our lives like a tsunami, undetected until it was nearly too late.

The wave of illness continues to ripple on the landscape of our lives. It is, however, now only the consequences of the backwash we are dealing with. The threat of death has been abated, at least temporarily. This is not our first encounter with the power of disease or injury. Life has given us several introductions to our mortality. Perhaps the practice has equipped us to navigate yet another unknown.

We have both survived poor prognoses more than once, most often with the unquestionable support of our health care providers and occasionally, in spite of them. Allen had open heart quadruple bypass surgery in 1981 followed by "heart events" off and on over the years. In 1996, he had prostate cancer surgery. He faced recurrence in 1998. Then in 2008, the lymphoma appeared.

I am myself no stranger to ill health. I remember those haunting words spoken by a compassionate physician in 1978 at my bedside while I was at St. Mary's Hospital (associated with the Mayo Clinic) . "We hope we have given you a year." I have not been consistently symptom free but can say, with considerable satisfaction, I am healthier in my sixties than I was at thirty. In other words, we are veterans of illness.

It was also to our benefit that I have spent much of my professional career in the service of those who experience chronic and life-threatening illness. However, being a clinician, and later a researcher addressing quality of life issues for those populations is a different journey than living the uncertainty of illness as the spouse of a very ill person.

Early in Allen's cancer experience, in the twilight of a late night in a hospital room, we agreed that the common metaphor, the war metaphor, didn't fit for us. The common expression about 'fighting cancer' was simply not Allen, simply not me, simply not us. Cancer was not "the enemy". There was no battle to win or lose. Cancer just was. Allen had done nothing to bring it on. In fact, his life style was commendable. He was a trim,

Zen and the Art of Illness

non-smoking vegetarian, happily married, and endeared to many. We chose the metaphor of "pilgrimage" which, by definition, is a journey undertaken knowing there are challenges and having an inner and outer destination. *Journey* literally means the distance travelled in one day.

Illness presents us with the reality of our impermanence. Serious or life-threatening illness does not allow the privilege of denying that we never come to an end. Although not steeped in the Buddhist tradition, I have been exposed to the precepts and practices of Soto Zen. The essence of Zen, as I understand it, is living in the moment, being present in the moment, living neither yesterday nor tomorrow. Living neither in fear, nor in hope, and yet, not without hope. As I look back, I realize that our response was to surrender to the moment. It was to do our best to simply be there in the moment, to do what needed to be done, to notice and respect whatever feelings arose. To accept each emotion as information, as an inner message to be acknowledged but not to be fueled. The gift for both of us was a deepened awareness of what it means to be human, what it means to suffer, what it means to be in relationship, and what it means to be whole.

We did our best to live without delusion, not to buffer the reality with beliefs we don't hold. On any given day, we understood our journey together could come to an end.

Zen and the Art of Illness

Speak your truth humbly

Phil Cousineau in his classic, *The Art of Pilgrimage*, notes that one of the traditions of pilgrimage is that one leaves something for the next pilgrim. Cousineau also suggests that "when in doubt, write."

Multitudes of people traverse the landscape of life-threatening illness each year. Perhaps there will be a moment recorded about our journey that will resonate, perhaps even help, another pilgrim weather a storm, survive a drought, ford a turbulent stream. Sharing our experience is, however, not without its risks.

Illness is a subjective experience lived on a personal landscape. The story of our pilgrimage was not documented day by day but as a reflection. I write subjectively about what was lived very personally. The excerpts are written in first person singular. It is the way the moments were lived, as if I am retelling, to Allen, the story of our journey as I lived it.

What any of us remember of our journey is recorded in our memories as moments, a series of snapshots or short videos. To describe the remembered moments is risky. It risks being known in ways that one may not have previously made visible. It risks implying and declaring unspoken pain. It risks saying how things seemed from the coordinates of one person's life. It risks attending to that which is often undervalued, even white washed. It risks offending someone whose part is perceived by them differently than it is recorded and indeed, it may have been. The greatest risk is to imply that the journey of one pilgrim is in any way to be an expectation of that of another pilgrim.

The telling of our story is intended only to share what we remember, the moments that stand out for us, particularly for me. It is not intended to teach or to interpret, to judge, or to even to praise. The landscape of illness has many peaks and valleys. Our narrative is more about the terrain, how we navigated the landscapes, how it changed over time and the people who were the human inukshuks we encountered as we traversed. Even for the few we met on a less than laudable day, we are grateful for their positive intent. And although our healthcare system has occasion for improvement, we applaud our access to it, and the care and competence of the many who encourage its maximum effort.

PRE-DIAGNOSIS:
Waiting in uncertainty

Strong and healthy,
who thinks of sickness
until it strikes like lightning?

UJetsum Milarepa (1052-1135)

Waiting in uncertainty

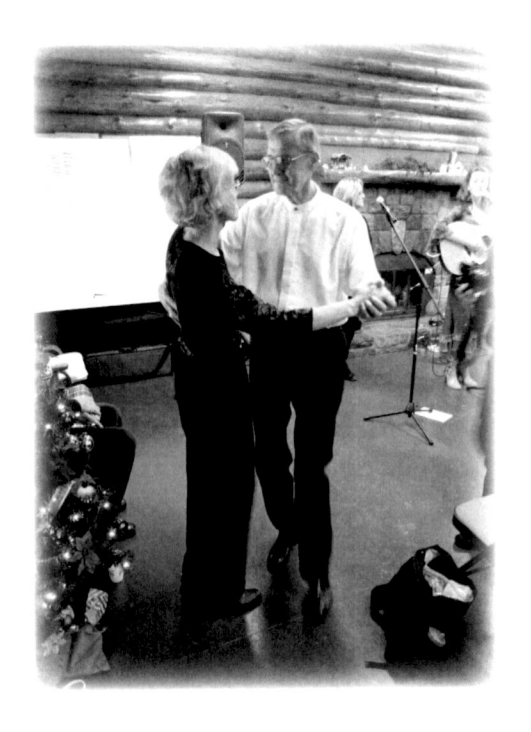

Zen and the Art of Illness

When I planned a three-day celebration for your 75th birthday, I didn't know that we would need an abundance of love in our hearts to face the yet unannounced storm.

They came from far and near, left their families to be with you on your special day, December 25, 2007. Even the weather cooperated. Shirtsleeve weather on Christmas Day. A hundred and ten came for the Boxing Day concert. We danced as Lizzy played "Can I have this dance for the rest of my life?" Friends and family applauded.

Somehow, we both feel safer between flannel sheets. Perhaps they bring back memories of being tucked in as a child. Dawn has brought us a blue pair. With flannels, you seem to get the chills less. They absorb more of the perspiration. We have only one pair. They are soaked by 2:00 a.m. each morning. By 5:a.m., those and another set of cotton sheets are washing. Somehow, the logic of purchasing a second set of flannels evades us.

Zen and the Art of Illness

The night sweats are flushing the energy from you with greater vengeance each night as the condition becomes more and more visible. Our eyes search each other's for evidence of assurance. It evades us. The moment calls for dry linens and fresh bedclothes. We fade into our next brief sleep to the sound of the washer. Hours later, the scenario repeats itself. Do I still go to the conference? We have an appointment at the doctors on Monday. This is Friday.

We didn't understand the night sweats. The raging drenching night sweats that took only moments were your body crying. Crying for help. Trying its best to help itself. At this point, it is all so foreign. We decide. I will keep my commitment to a major speaking engagement in Victoria.

Zen and the Art of Illness

It's hard being a thousand miles away lecturing about hope and palliative care, not knowing how you are. Calling home every two hours. Being on constant alert. We are both sensing something is seriously wrong. Your weight is dropping. Your energy is almost non-existent. Your appetite is minimal. Every test has been negative. But something is wrong. We sense it. Our physician concurs. But what? It is like life has been put on hold with a pause button.

Waiting in uncertainty

The winds blow as they rarely blow. Thank goodness the plane could land. Why did there have to be a storm tonight. In 14 years, we have only had to plough out our lane twice. A prairie blizzard is a thing to be reckoned with. A white-out means trusting your instinct that the road is still there. It means taking cues from the little glimpses of the road that become visible. Thank goodness for nephews. Brett's heavy truck is enough to get me up the long driveway that was fast succumbing to the heavy snowfall. When though could we next get out? When would the storm subside? It is not the only storm awaiting me.

Zen and the Art of Illness

Your fever is 103 degrees. Your voice faint. I call Helplink. I stay on the line for an hour listening to the periodic recording, "We value your call. One of our agents will be with you shortly. Please stay on the line and your call will be answered in the order …" The nurses who answer the Helplink phones couldn't get in for their shifts.

There is no point in calling an ambulance. They wouldn't be able to get up the lane. EMS can't get in. We can't get out. Using my cell phone, I wake up my friend Alice - nurse Alice, nurse administrator Alice, but mostly our friend, Alice.

With her guidance, we lower your temperature. I speak soothingly. We both know that the situation is serious. The fever continues but it doesn't climb. Somehow, we will get out in the morning.

It will take a monster truck to get us out. Jan (Dutch for John) agrees to come. His four-wheel drive with a raised suspension makes it up the hill. Jan and I confer. We will all go out in the monster truck together. The drifts are such that I would not be able to follow by car. We are on our way to help. Stay calm.

You insist on street clothes. Changing you exhausts both of us. You hang on limply as Jan hoists you into the vehicle. We clasp the seat belt for you as you flop toward the headrest. A strange silence goes unbroken. It is Monday morning. The journey has begun.

Zen and the Art of Illness

Dr. Jeffrey has you admitted immediately. Blood work, x-rays, the parade of welcome invasions. You drift in and out of sleep. Drenched and changed. Drenched and changed. Too weary for fear.

Somehow the biopsy is to happen that very day. Someone will make it happen. They confirm the biopsy will happen. You will be sedated. Knowing that, you ask to sit up, ask for a pen, and you write a holograph will. Only weeks ago, we had begun revamping our complicated will. In one sentence, you simplify it.

We wait. Three days. Inconclusive. It is Thursday. A more invasive approach will be necessary. We wait again. Wait for the call to be transferred to a major hospital in the city. They will do thoracic surgery to attempt diagnosis. Four days pass.

There is a morsel of peace of mind in the holograph will. In the insuing days, the revisions to the will that we began weeks before are not forthcoming. Somehow the urgency evades our lawyer. Every phone call provides a lame explanation and a new promise for a quick response, as if pleasantness is a substitute for efficiency. I have to let go of trying to make it happen. I simply call every few days. I work into the conversation the seriousness of your condition. The investments are tanking by the day. Is the will even realistic?

I cannot look outward for certainty in any area of life right now. The combination of issues are fodder for anxiety. I need to not go there. I can't re-do life and suddenly have a pension. I can't fix the economy, and I can't fix your condition. I have to co-habit with uncertainty.

Zen and the Art of Illness

Aware that I need sleep, I leave you in the care of strangers at night. I am aware that I can best serve you if I am somewhat rested, when my mind is eased by paid bills and cancelled agendas. It is hard to hear that a night nurse was annoyed that she had to change your linens and bedclothes. That she offered no solace. That she tended your body and left your soul to ache. That she treated you like an inconvenience.

It is harder to leave the next night. Harder to trust. I resolve to stay at your side more nights.

The call comes Monday morning. The ambulance attendants prepare to transfer you to the city. As you leave, we have that brief moment. You have that little smile that tells me you are in the moment. That it is okay for me to go home and collect what I need for the unknown time frame that I will be away. That you know we are doing this together. That you will not be alone. That I will be there for you. That brief silent moment comforts both of us. I head home and am on my way again within the hour.

I wonder how young mothers and elderly wives do this. I have no dog to feed, no childcare to arrange, no work setting that demands my presence.

Zen and the Art of Illness

Every volunteer who has ever served an hour in a hospital gift shop has given more than they might ever imagine. Hospital gift shops are the smallest supermarkets on the planet. From snacks to cards, from lighthearted gifts to the practical necessities of being caught in unexpected waiting, the gift shop will have something that will work. In your case, the slippers with the velcro tabs are perfect. They have your size. There is something hopeful about getting you new slippers.

We wait. The waiting extends to three days. Three days on the emergency surgery wait list. We live the oxymoron. Three days that you cannot have food or drink. At eleven each night, you are allowed to drink, and we start over in the morning. At 8 p.m.. on the third night, Dr. Stewart compassionately agrees to come in specifically to do the thoracic surgery. You are weaker than when you were transferred. I pace in the twilight of the solarium as I wait. With its greenery, the ambience could be mistaken for the shore of a tropical seaside. No lapping of the waves though. Just the pounding of "what ifs" on the shores of our future.

Zen and the Art of Illness

I pace while you are in surgery. I call Susan. I explain where I am and what is happening. I explain that I simply need to tell someone. I have no expectation of her being able to do anything. I just need the sound of another person's voice, a voice that I know has worked in the context I am now in. A voice that would know what *not* to say. Someone who would know to just listen. Someone who would know that there are no words designed for the occasion.

Dr. Stewart speaks in a gentle direct manner. He is suspicious of lymphoma. He will ask for the results, STAT. We should know in a couple of days.

We wait. Five days. The weekend. Yes ,of course, a weekend. Disease must stop for weekends. You are allowed to return home for this wait. You are fading in increments.

Zen and the Art of Illness

It is good to be home while we await the results. I call homecare and am pleased with a promise of a quick response. We wait. Two and a half days. The assessment takes place on Saturday morning. The supervisor details your condition, extends compassion, notes the extent of your incapacities, and assures us someone will be there Monday morning.

We wait. Tuesday you stagger; you are very unstable as I assist you to the bathroom. I can't support you sufficiently. We both fall. I am the one injured. It is weeks before my back recovers. I must find a rightful place for the resentment that the system cannot provide what it truly intends to.

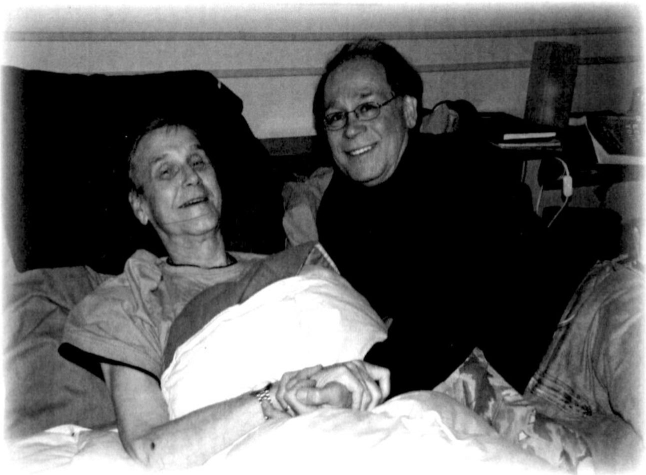

Zen and the Art of Illness

It is Wednesday. Still no homecare. None of the promised equipment. Yes, we are cleared for everything. Just - the new occupational therapist isn't oriented yet, and there isn't any staff to send to help with a bath.

Two calls. One to Nels, my brother, and in many ways, your brother. He is nearby. One to John, our good friend. Yes, of course, he will come forty miles to help give you the only thing you have asked for in weeks. A bath. John climbs onto the bed and consults with you directly. In a few minutes, he and Nels will place you on the bath chair left from Dad's last years. John has stripped to his shorts and is in the bathtub while Nels more or less lifts you in and onto the stool. Nels has rigged a hose to the showerhead. John shampoos your head. You are exhausted but pleased. You are asleep minutes after they have you back in bed.

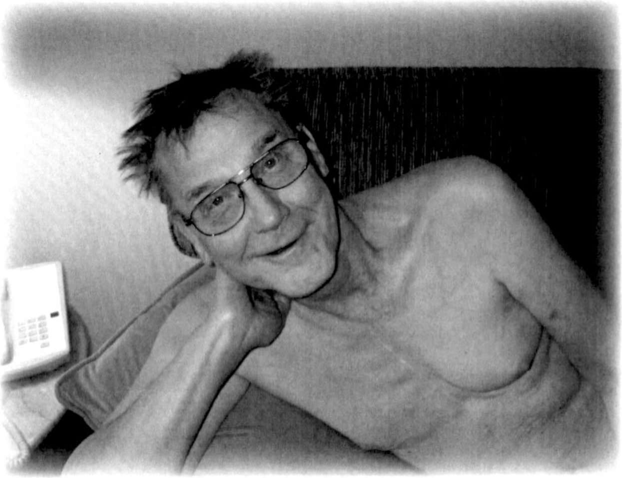

Zen and the Art of Illness

Perhaps it is a good thing you can't see yourself. Can't see your collarbone protruding like that of a concentration camp prisoner.

Dr. Jeffery calls. It is nearly seven. She is still at work. She shares that the tentative diagnosis has been confirmed. More tests coming. Someone from the cancer hospital will phone in the morning. Morning comes and the male voice says, "Is Mr. Eng available?" I share, "Mr. Eng is ill. Can I help you?" The male voice replies, "This is Dr. Reiman. I was thinking I might be able to help." Our affable exchange turns to the real issue. You will be admitted as soon as a bed is available. If not today, then tomorrow. We wait. The call comes at noon the next day.

IN-PATIENT:

Living in a medical culture

"I am here" is a practice.

Thich Nhat Hahn.

Nels is waiting for my call. He will help me get you into the car. He isn't answering his cell. He has forgotten to turn it on after a meeting. I know where Nels is. He is only five minutes away. I will get him. But he isn't there. Dawn, my sister-in-law, who is home, returns with me. So does Angel, their young Mexican friend. He takes his cue from Dawn. Time is collapsed. Everything is now. Not in a rushed way. In a still way. Dawn has reached Nels. He will be here in minutes.

A ten-minute absence has been too long. You tried to move yourself and fell to the floor. You are sprawled, lifeless on the bedroom floor. As we enter, you turn your head, acknowledging the helplessness. There are no words. Angel looks at me, and all three of us engage in the awkward task of getting you onto the edge of the bed. There are issues of dignity that none of us address directly. The eyes that used to sparkle are hollow.

As Nels lifts you into the car, snaps you in, and closes the door, he and I lock glances. He shakes his head gently. No words. We both understand. You are likely leaving home forever.

The hour drive is quiet. It hasn't occurred to me to trust you to an ambulance. To let you leave, perhaps more logically, more comfortably, in an ambulance. To let you go alone. It is perhaps my need for you to know, you will not do this alone.

I stop at the front desk. Marie is there. After 25 years, she is still at the front desk, still pleasant, still so obliging. Still calling me Dr. Jevne. I share that I have you in the car, that I will need help in the ambulance bay. She agrees to send a physiotherapist quickly to assist. I already have your door open when the physio arrives. Obviously, she is expecting someone more ambulatory, more able to help themselves. She hesitates, then says, "I will just be a moment". Someone joins her, and the transfer to a wheelchair is done with precision.

Zen and the Art of Illness

The blur of admission begins. You slip in and out of what seems like sleep. The pokes and prods come and go. You are too weary to answer all but essential questions. You cooperate with everything and question nothing. It is the way of the system. It saves your life by taking it.

My presence is felt. I am silent. Sitting quietly in your presence. Finding that place between retired professional and wife. Presenting myself as companion and yet clearly the gatekeeper to your life. A delicate balance. We are here and, at least at this point, what can be done, what must be done, is being done.

You are here, but you aren't here. The organism in the bed hardly seems like the Allen either of us know. I am fully aware, or as aware as I am capable of, that the organism may die. It seems so wrong that you may die on Valentine's Day.

Zen and the Art of Illness

Doug is sitting in the chair when I enter the room. His elbows are supported on his knees, his head is resting in his palms. His eyes search mine. We both know there are no words. In his gentle way, he says, "And I thought I had a bad day with students." He admits that he had no idea that you were as ill as you are.

In the ensuing months, he is there for you. A phone call here. A visit there. He always brings a movie for the two of you to watch once you are home. And two specialty beers, one for each of you every time he comes. It's a one hour drive but he finds the time. He takes the time. Often, you are too weary for conversation, and yet no visit is more welcome.

Years ago, I sat in committee meetings advocating for the unit of care to be the patient <u>and</u> the family, and for there to be 24 hour visiting privileges. Today, that means I am offered the opportunity to sleep on a roll out cot in your room. What I didn't realize is, it would be on the same cot offered patient and family members 25 years ago! I use two flannel sheets to disguise the protruding springs and am grateful to drift off in the twilight that is night in a hospital room. I say nothing of the discomfort. I lie with my head across from your feet. We exchange a silent smile and both drift off.

Zen and the Art of Illness

I am surprised how soundly I have slept. Yet, like the mother of a newborn, I am startled to wakefulness with an awareness of your rousing. You are drenched. I push the call button, and help is almost instantaneous. With the touch that comes from compassion combined with experience, the words comfort, and the bed is changed efficiently. The soaked pajamas are exchanged and assurances given. And I know we are safe. As safe as it is possible to be. We both slip back into needed sleep.

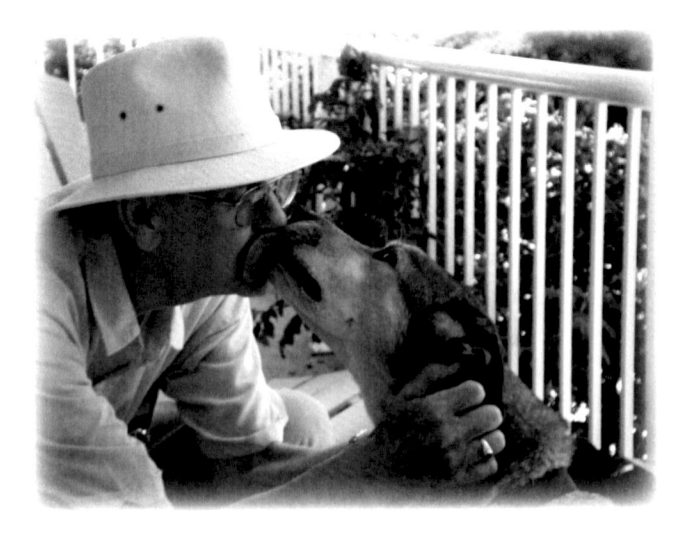

Zen and the Art of Illness

The dream was vivid. It was so real. I wasn't even sure I was asleep, but I must have been. We were both almost glad that we weren't at home when Molly had to be put down last summer. The cancer got her. Thirteen is a ripe age for a large dog, but still it was hard to authorize the decision.

I remember the last time you cupped her face in your hands and gave her a kiss as we left on a trip not knowing if we would ever see her again. In the dream, she lay beside your bed, her front legs outstretched. Clearly, she was guarding you. At the end of the bed was a lone wolf, standing but not aggressively. Clearly, Molly and the wolf had an understanding. The wolf would come no closer. No Freudian interpretation needed. Molly was doing what she could to keep the wolf at the door at bay.

The choice for chemotherapy will depend on the assessment of your heart's capacity to tolerate it. It is 27 years since your quadruple open-heart by-pass surgery. The hospital across the city has information on your heart from the pre-op for the diagnostic surgery. They agree to send it on Monday. It is Friday noon. That means no treatment until after the weekend. The unit clerk, the staff physician, and the head nurse are conferring as I stand at the desk for an innocuous request. I sense their frustration with bureaucracy. I understand that Allen may not have until Monday. I volunteer to get the test results. Reluctantly, I leave you. Three hours later, I have the tracings in my hands. The head nurse smiles as she says, "You are good. You are good!" Little does she know the respect and the near groveling it took to get the information despite carrying a copy of your legal personal directive papers. My reply is a smile and a "Thank you." I return to your room. You are sleeping. I am quietly apprehensive. Will they treat?

Zen and the Art of Illness

We have met the staff physician. He is calling the shots, ordering the tests, explaining things the best he can. He is direct yet pleasant. He leaves no doubt that things are serious. It is twenty-seven hours before we meet your oncologist. He is quiet spoken. He also leaves no doubt that things are serious and that treatment will be tough. This is the first indication that we have had that there will be treatment. With whispered words and a gesture, you defer to me after ensuring Dr. Reiman understands that I am the agent of your personal directive.

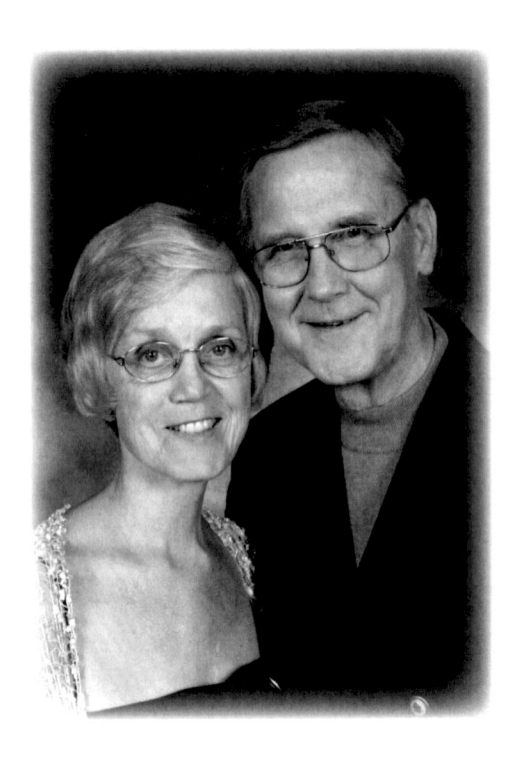

Zen and the Art of Illness

Above your bed, I have hung a photograph of us taken not long ago. I ask Dr. Reiman to look at it and to understand that you looked like that recently. He smiles and acknowledges that our family physician has already called him and firmly asserted that this man is much younger and healthier than his medical record would suggest. He declares, based on that, he is willing to take somewhat more risk. We don't know exactly what that means, but we know that means that there is a chance. There is at least a chance. Chemotherapy will start tomorrow. I express my surprise that chemo will start on a Saturday. The words I hear are no surprise. "We may not have until Monday."

That night the drenching reoccurs. Twice by 2 a.m. You are not able to drift back to sleep. I crawl up onto the bed, cradle your weak body in my arms, and you drift off with your head on my shoulder. Eventually, I slip off the bed and back onto the cot from hell.

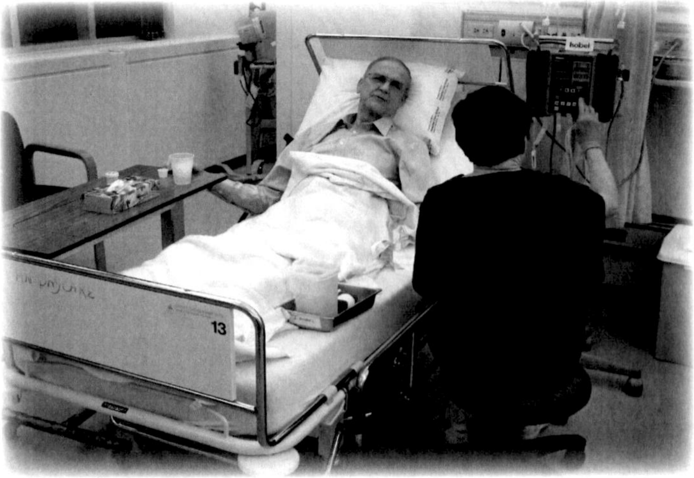

Zen and the Art of Illness

She is young and yet experienced. The intravenous stand has multiple plastic bags hanging from it. Six, if I remember. Despite your weariness, she engages you in conversation. Once she has prepared the area, she takes your left forearm, looks you in the eye and says, "Are we ready?" Your reply is, "As ready as I can be I guess." With a little smile you add, "Do you mean other than being scared to death?" You share it with a smile but she hears the true intent. We are both amazed when she gently says, "Well then, we aren't ready. We need to talk a while. Can you tell me more about what you are afraid of?" Somehow within minutes, she gains your confidence and treatment begins. It will take eight hours to infuse the six drugs.

Unknown to you, I have permission from your roommate who is dying of colon cancer for a little surprise. An hour after chemo has begun, Maya appears. She has driven 75 miles to appear in your room. You are so dear to her. She is in her crimson velvet performance gown, and her violin is tucked under her arm. She simply smiles at you, greets you with only a word or two, and begins to play. If there are angels, she is one of them. The chemo nurse is as moved as you are. The whole focus shifts to this personal concert that is less than fifteen minutes but will be a lifetime memory. She slips away as mystically as she appeared. I regret that I don't have my camera. The image is forever captured on our souls.

Zen and the Art of Illness

I awoke startled. And angry. Strange, waking up angry. I rearranged the pillow to support my back as I sat up. Time passed. I sat with the anger. Just sat with it. Didn't fuss at it. Didn't fuss with it. Just sat with it. Eventually the words, even though sub-vocal, come forward with strength. "I am not doing a memorial! I am just not doing one! I already did a huge birthday, and I am not doing another event. I am not great with large groups. It takes a lot of planning. I am not doing it." That settles it. You have to survive because I am not doing a memorial! I inform you in the morning, and you agree. We both smile. We both know I that I might be doing a memorial.

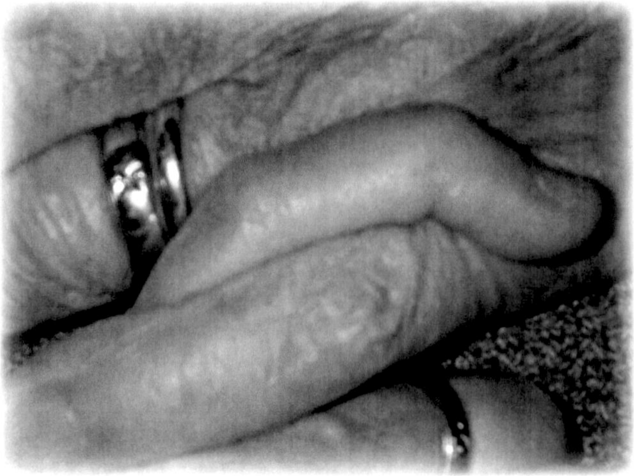

Zen and the Art of Illness

The advances in anti-nausea medication are a godsend. Chemo number one has gone well. That night the drenching sweats return. With dry linens and pajamas, you await sleep. It doesn't come. The prednisone is likely contributing to the insomnia. At 2:30 a.m. in the twilight of the room, I sit on your bedside. You haven't eaten anything all day. You agree to try a little soy chocolate pudding. As I slip the first teaspoon into your mouth, you have that trademark little smile. You consume only mouthfuls of the little carton. We hook little fingers, and we know we are doing this together. No words are required.

For a moment, I thought David was coming to visit us. Just as I realized he was headed for the next unit, his eye caught mine. It seems his sister was diagnosed with the same condition as you have. Things though have gone wrong. He is here with his mother who is likely having a last visit with her daughter. Her daughter was considered much lower risk than you. She will die the following day of complications of treatment. She is twenty years your junior. Do I tell you? I choose silence.

Zen and the Art of Illness

There are long hours of silence. I am not drawn to the lounge or to conversations with those who come and go, professional or volunteer. The afternoon tea is nice though, a few moments of being pampered. The sensitive host doesn't extract the price of social trivia for attending. I am reminded of my fridge magnet, "Where there is tea, there is hope."

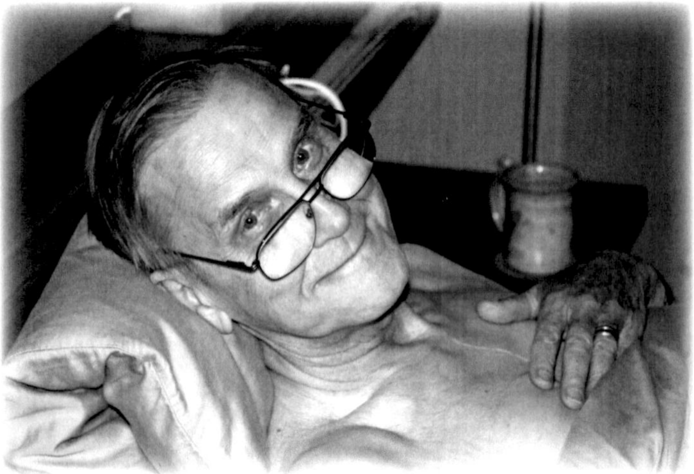

Zen and the Art of Illness

Word travels fast. There are very few visitors for days. The grapevine has accurately conveyed how ill you are. Those who come stay only minutes. The reality of your condition is not blind to anyone. In several days though, you are able to support your upper body slightly, you are again present in your eyes, and your trademark smile has reappeared. We dare to hope.

There is something about male visitors. They don't talk about illness in terms of feelings. They exchange information. They give an update about the outside world, perhaps share a little humor, and leave an expectation that they intend to see you improving soon. When a man leaves, it is like he leaves part of his strength in the room, leaves a kind of masculine energy of some kind that is exchanged only between men. I wonder if they know how important their visits were to both of us. How their visits said something, something that could not be said with anything but their presence.

Zen and the Art of Illness

The days drift into more days. My own energy is being diluted with boredom and endless sedentary steadfastness. The hospital is a good host. I am offered a shower but choose to go to friends who live nearby. I can go and be back in an hour. Not that there is any hurry but I am not looking for chit-chat. Silence is actually comforting. Routine is comforting. I calculate how many times I need to walk around the unit so that I am walking at least a kilometer before bed each night.

I am sedentary during the day. My presence means that you will get the sip of water when you are thirsty. You will have the advocate every patient needs when there is a miscommunication among professionals or with us. It means you will never be cold and never feel abandoned. It means you can sleep peacefully knowing I am only a few feet away or in the lounge next door. It means I can feel my body growing weary without normal rest and normal exercise. I am a basically a kinesthetic person. I need to move. It is simply my nature.

Zen and the Art of Illness

It seems like a strange time to decide to learn to swim. I can already dog paddle a bit. Swimming can't be that hard. I am not afraid of water, and there is a pool not far away. I have recently had an ear surgery that means I can submerge my head (not far) below the water. It seems like a perfectly logical thing to do - learn to swim while your husband is going through life-threatening treatment. Seems reasonable! I just begin. Somehow, opportunities to be away for an hour here and there present themselves.

The morning that I stayed nearby at Don and Bev's, I had a shower and a good night's sleep. I returned to find you looking weak and pale. You reported that you had fallen. In the ensuing hour, the nurse wants you to rise for your morning ritual, the physiotherapist arrives to assist with your morning walk, and home care arrives to make final arrangements for you to go home.

No one seems to know that you had fallen. The fall has apparently not been documented. Therefore, somehow the fall hasn't happened. You assure your nurse, accompanied with your trademark smile, that indeed, you had fallen. The bruising, if not present now, would be ample evidence soon. My request to have the fall recorded is met with a defensive, "It won't affect my nursing". I assured the nurse we had not meant any ill intent but that it was information that might be relevant to the discharge planning, physiotherapy, and homecare. Again, with milder defensiveness, the response was hesitancy. My final plea was cloaked in humor as I repeated the request to document the fall. I suggested that she add that the patient's spouse is a cranky woman who wanted the fall during the night documented. I assure her, that I would accept full responsibility for her doing what was seemingly not required.

Zen and the Art of Illness

A visit from the head nurse pleasantly informs us that, indeed, the fall had been recorded as an incident report and had been taken seriously. However, when an incident report is done, policy dictates that it goes directly to administration. She reported that the "hole in the system" would be closed with new policy that would include documenting the incident in the progress notes as well. We are simply pleased that the physiotherapist reassessed you and that you were sent to x-ray to check for a cracked rib. And that a win-win was possible. We truly love win-wins.

Ceinwen and Marilyn find us in a waiting room on the lower floor waiting for the x-ray. Marilyn is head of the Arts and Medicine Program at the hospital and is as gentle as they make people. Ceinwen, a small Welsh woman I have known for years, is also one of the psychologists. She is as kind as they make people. With their experience, they know enough to stay only minutes. They present you with a teddy bear. That little smile slips on to your countenance, and Teddy is still with us today.

Zen and the Art of Illness

Around two weeks had passed since your admission, and there were rumblings about us possibly going home. Then, we found out that those discussions had stopped hours ago and that you were being moved into semi-isolation based on new blood test results. The fact that you were also so weak from a fall, had not yet circulated to the various services.

As the mini-lecture on the role of discharge planning poured out without the slightest intent to inquire about our needs, I had to call on my best Zen self not to openly smile. It did help that a veteran nurse, who was present, was cringing as maturely as one could cringe while still being professional. My comment was, "I share your concern that we go home with things in place". I said this respectfully, unlike the the tone of the nurse's lecturette. I was committed to neither alienate anyone who could help, nor would I grovel or worship at the temple of the obvious. My effort at respectful communication came not from a place of fear but rather from a deep respect for positive intent. A later encounter had none of the patronizing overtones. I hesitate to hypothisize the reason for the shift in her approach.

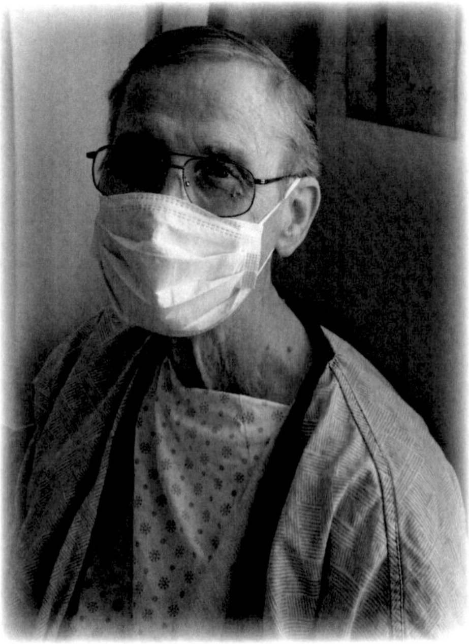

Zen and the Art of Illness

We thought we would be going home today. Another surprise. Your counts have dropped dramatically, into dangerously low levels. Your immune system has crashed. There are lots of technical terms. We understand that you will start a series of shots daily to counter the problem. We behave rather unemotionally, as if we have heard that our flight has been rescheduled. There is no energy left for radical hope or false despair.

Given your blood counts, the ward physician wants you in semi isolation. By nightfall, the transfer hasn't happened despite us knowing there is a room available, actually more than one. I am able to decipher through the night nurse that we are the fallout of a mild turf war. Who decides what? I sit for a full hour meditating so that I can navigate the dilemma with respect rather than the aggressiveness that tends to arise as a first response when I think you are threatened. The outcome though must be that you are moved to the new room. It happens and no one loses face.

Zen and the Art of Illness

On my walk before bed, I talk to myself. Don't get attached to expectations. Don't get attached to when things are going to happen or who is responsible for making them happen. Amazingly compassionate things happen unexpectedly, and minor omissions and conflicts happen in the day-to-day workings of hospitalization. Things change from day to day. Don't get attached to hope. Don't dismiss it. Just don't get attached to it. Don't get attached to despair. Don't dismiss it. Just don't get attached to it. Don't get attached to outcomes or labels.

Remember what David Ricco says in *Five Things We Cannot Change.* Things end, and things change, and things don't always go according to plan. Life is not always fair, and pain is part of life. I get it - but it isn't always easy.

We are vegan. That means that we don't eat animal products. We do consume a little fish for the omega three oils. As you begin to have a little interest in eating, we ask to see the dietician. Despite indicating that we understand the limits of food services to cater to special needs or preferences, we are met with what we experience as defensiveness. We find it odd that it is us who are putting staff at ease. It becomes clear that our genuine respect is not immediately assessed as such. Once our young nutritionist acknowledges our intent, the conversation turns into quiet exchanges. Soymilk will not be available for cereal. We do learn that if we provide two days notice, there actually are some vegetarian meals available. We express our gratitude for whatever is possible.

Zen and the Art of Illness

Planet Organic is a godsend. Ten minutes from the hospital, I can purchase vegan foods. The little fridge in the refreshment room on the ward keeps things cool. I mark our food but there is little chance someone will be craving our tofu scramble. I prepare almost all of your meals, little as they are. We are grateful for the morning porridge and supplement it with almond milk.

In a moment of lightness, I kid you. "Honey, don't worry about the cancer. The food will kill ya'." Your eyes smile. What would I do without that smile? We both know food is not the real issue, at least not for a while. I go daily and bring back anything that I think might entice you to eat, even a little.

The bed-chair that is in your new private room far exceeds the comfort of the cot in the first room. I actually sleep several hours at a time. We are alone in the room, and the gift of privacy is a welcome change.

Zen and the Art of Illness

I learn to glove and mask. I am taught to give you injections. I will need to do so ten out of twenty days once we leave the hospital. With a brother who was diabetic and as someone who injects my own B12, I am not squeamish. Over the ensuing months, I will take pride in producing less bruising than nursing staff inflicted.

I decide to keep my appointment with Dr. Cherry. For 15 years she has watched over my condition. I see her routinely every three months regardless of my health status. For the most part, my condition is well controlled. I am more vulnerable under duress. She is one of those rare physicians who ask about your whole life in a non-intrusive way. She has that rare quality of simply listening and inquiring. I told her of the seriousness of your condition. As I leave her office, she looks up from her five-foot slender frame and says quietly, almost tentatively, "I am Catholic. I will say a prayer." Why is it that some people can say that and it feels like a gift while from others, it feels intrusive? From her, it is a gift.

Zen and the Art of Illness

The cell phone rings a few times a day. Later the bill says just how many times. $512.00 worth in one month. I learn that we are paying for incoming calls. I switch plans.

The well wishes are appreciated. I am not always comfortable with the unsolicited advice and the rare, but unforgettable, declarations that we need to pray harder. Somehow that doesn't seem how this works. I have never been convinced that prayer is a mail order catalogue for my personal wishes. In my own way, I find the strength and patience to be there for you as you have always been there for me.

There are those words again, "You must be so afraid." I wonder how many times I have heard them. Each time I respond with some kind of tactical diversion. I have no direct response. I remember a story I read about a Jewish physician awaking to the Gestapo pounding on his front door. He turned to his wife and said, "The time for fear has passed. The time for hope has begun."

I never share the story with those who offer their version of empathy. How could I justify not being afraid? Afraid of what? No-one ever says. I suppose that they mean afraid of you dying. This situation warrants more from me than fear. Living from a place of fear is not going to help. How can I explain that I am more afraid of the system failing us, of some petty policy interfering with your treatment than of the reality of death? More afraid of what is within someone's control, than what is in no one's control. Being afraid feels like making this experience more about me than about you. The last thing you need is a wife living from a place of fear. Maybe I just don't do fear very well.

OUT-PATIENT:
In limbo, but home

There is something healing
in watching your own roses bloom.

Ronna Jevne

We are not new to "cancer diet" perspectives. We have been vegan for years. Somehow though, we intensify our efforts. We are guided by the recent reading of *The China Study*. I purge the pantry and the fridge of anything obviously a violation of the discipline we intend. The dark chocolate though stays! Your appetite is minimal. I am in a search pattern for alternatives to keep your weight from dropping further. I make my first avocado shake. Juice of two lemons. Juice of one lime. Half of a long cucumber, one avocado. Eight ice cubes. A cup of soymilk. Blend the blazes out of it. I take it into you offering it with the words, "Anything this color can't taste good." You smile and take a sip. As your eyebrows rise as a sign of the tartness, you nod approvingly. Over time, we learn to add a few drops of stevia.

Zen and the Art of Illness

The needles seem endless. There are needles for this, and needles for that, and needles that are given twice a day, and needles that are three times a day for 10 days out of every 20. There's blood thinner and there's an injection to help counter your suppressed immune system. Your abdominal area looks like a battleship torpeodoed once too many! I am grateful for being raised with a diabetic. As a child, I learned, when necessary, to give an injection to my brother Tom. The community health nurse had Nels and I practice on oranges. As a child, I thought it was fun. In my adult life, I had given my own bi-weekly injection for years. Somehow, it is not as easy to give you the five shots a day you need. However, being willing to do so means we can be home.

I invent the frog. We never name him. I tell stories about him living in a swamp. He has adventures. He has friends. He distracts you from the impending injection. We smile. Then the frog leaps, and the injection is over. Months later, during one of the pre-injection times, I ask you, "Where is the frog?" You smile, and with a boyish look reply, "He is hiding under a lily pad. He doesn't want a needle." I play with the bedclothes, find the lily pad and poof - the frog leaps, the injection happens.

Zen and the Art of Illness

Other than the incident of the frog, neither of us have been able to recall any memory that we would call a funny moment, let alone something over which we have had a belly laugh. I guess that says it all. It wasn't that we were without humor. The gift, as time passes, is that we are more able to see the irony in some things. It warms my heart to hear you tell the story of the day we took you to the Cross. You can get people laughing about how you fell out of bed and couldn't move yourself, let alone get back into the bed. That's truly perspective.

Some things are just too painful. They can be contained in privacy or in a very small group, but Easter dinner with thirty people will be too much. I know I can't handle "How's Allen?", the many times it would be asked. I know that I can't bring any joy, not even emotional neutrality, to a family function. The week has been hard. I am not willing to leave you even for an hour, even for the conversations I need, the laughter I miss. I make my share of the meal and send it over. It is hard eating alone. Hard missing all those desserts! Besides the difficult logistics of slipping away for an hour or two, I know my heart is here at home. The loneliness of illness generates a hope that someone may bring over a desert. I question myself, "How often have I forgotten those who are absent?"

Zen and the Art of Illness

At first, I didn't recognize the voice. I hadn't heard it in twenty-four years. Through a circuitous route, she has heard of our situation. The call is simple, empathic and practical. She remains grateful for help that I extended years ago and conveys, "If there is anything, anything at all that I can do, please call". There is a warm place in my heart for her after all these years, a place she earned as she walked a similar walk. In those days, there wasn't much that could be done. She lost him. She knows the path we are walking.

Cathy has come to stay with him for a day to accommodate me attending an all day meeting in the city. At noon, the phone rings. He isn't doing well. I am only blocks from the hospital. When I am at home, we would call the triage nurse for guidance. My meeting is only a stone's throw from the cancer center. It seemed logical to just walk over and talk with somone.

Going to the hospital was almost comedic. You can only phone the triage nurse, not actually talk to her in person. So there I am! Calling her from the phone in the foyer, trying to accomplish the obvious while we talk through a closed door. Fate sometimes smiles at the right time. Your doctor, who the nurse reported was not in the hospital, notices me as he walks by (in his white coat and obviously on duty) and stops. In the caring and pleasant way we have come to expect of him, he inquires about what is happening. Even he smiles and shakes his head before asking a series of questions that within minutes lead to a clear, decisive direction. It is also quite clear that he and the triage nurse would be having a discussion! I urged gentleness. He smiled.

Zen and the Art of Illness

I know they have to charge for parking. At least, there is parking. Day after day the costs add up. Not a big consideration given that one of your shots is $212.00 a shot, and you need ten of them a month. Still, paying for parking feels like a tax on the ill. I wonder how some families manage the out of pocket expenses. We are grateful that we have additional insurance to pay part of the drug costs. How does the single working mom be there for an ill or dying family member?

Whether you survive or succumb, we will not be bankrupt to have given you a chance. A day doesn't pass without being grateful that our decisions are not based on means, at least not most of them. Tommy Douglas was voted by the Canadian people as the Greatest Canadian for having brought in universal health care. Because of his leadership and compassion, we are blessed as Canadians. We don't have to live in fear of uncertainty, without access to health care. We don't have to navigate a maze of insurance bureaucracy during a time already riddled with the pressures of illness. Surely as a nation, we can preserve this common sense reality of sharing the burden of the lack of good fortune. Every one of us is only a diagnosis away from being the brother, or sister, who needs keeping.

Zen and the Art of Illness

The disadvantage of living in a community where you know almost no one is that no casseroles arrive, no one calls to offer to get groceries, the mail gets picked up only when I get to it. If the microwave breaks down, it will have to stay that way for a while. Our emotional community is not geographically close. Bless Dawn for putting in the flowers and the garden. The earth might well have remained black for the summer without her tending. Nels is generous with his quiet gifts of time. There are occasional gestures by others whose worlds are full of their own demands. We are grateful for each of them.

Today's chemo nurse is a veteran, likely near retirement. She's chatty, excited about an upcoming overseas trip. There is no inquiry from her about your condition beyond the basics. The usual explanations are seemingly bypassed with the assumption that they are not needed. About half way through the day, we inquire about the redness that is developing, rather dramatically, on your vein. She assures us that it is a little more than normal but will be fine. We have insufficient experience to go beyond wondering if the infusion site should be moved. The words intended to reassure are somehow hollow. There is a sense of not being heard. You pay the price of us being right but not assertive. Within a day or two you are under treatment for a serious blood clot that extends from above the inside of your elbow to just below the your armpit. We are told it is now more immediately dangerous than the cancer. We put no energy into who is to blame. The issue is to deal with the complication. More shots. More scans. More appointments.

Zen and the Art of Illness

In our culture, perhaps in many, bladder control is about dignity. Your body can't concentrate on the smaller matters while it is trying to save your life. I admire your willingness to accept the realities of the moment. Not to apologize or resent what is presently outside of everyone's control. You are not your body. And you know the difference.

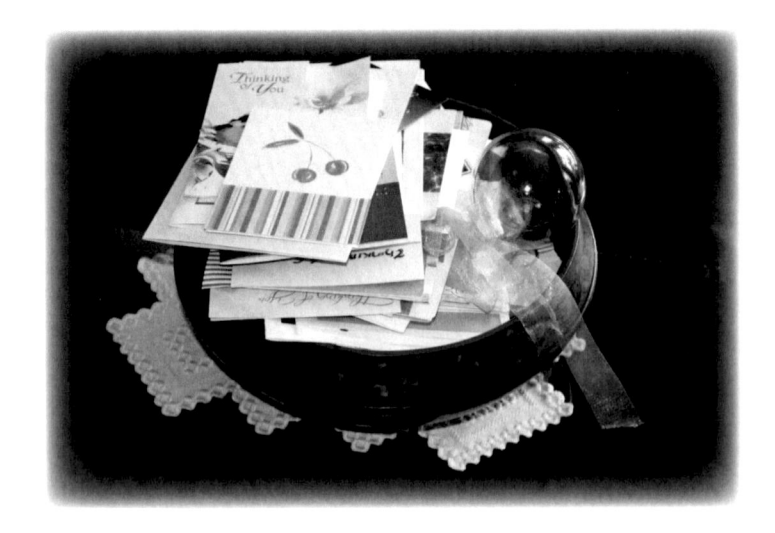

Zen and the Art of Illness

Over time, the stream of well wishes slip into the recesses of time like the floods of the spring slip into the dry creek beds of the summer. People go on with their lives. Rightly so. On the occasional day when someone invites us spontaneously for a luncheon, it is hard for both of us when we realize you simply cannot generate the energy to go. We comfort each other with the reality that declining an invitation is the wise choice, and we talk about the limits of the condition. We regret "the condition" has made our world smaller. The large bowl filled with cards reminds us there is a world awaiting us.

Five injections spaced out over the day. You are not stable enough to venture more than a few feet on your own. Thank goodness for the floor to ceiling pole that has been installed at your bedside. Some one comes for "bath assist" once a week but we are on our own for the remainder of the time. You sleep much of the day. There is almost always a high calorie shake on the bedside table, usually avocado, lemon, lime, cucumber and soy milk. You've grown fond of them. Life is doled out in half hour, at most one hour, stints. Anything that takes more than that has to be pre-planned. Home becomes a sanctuary. We work consciously for it not to become a prison.

Zen and the Art of Illness

The e-mail was brief. Kuya offered to come. I e-mailed back that there wasn't much anyone could do. She indicated if she came, that she would simply sit in silence outside of his door. Just by saying so, she was offering strength. I loved that she rang the temple bell for you.

It's hard wanting you to eat. Somehow there is a grandmother in me that feels that if you could just eat this, or that, you would get stronger. The hollow in your eyes would fill, and the darkness under them would give way to flesh tones. I need to remember that your mouth is ulcerated and your appetite, non-existent. You're good about trying a little blended soup, and you like the berry shakes. I make food preparation an art form based on what seems to make sense for someone so ill and that conforms to anti-cancer recommendations. I have no idea if it is actually helping you. I know it helps me. It helps me feel like we are doing what is within our control. On chemo graduation day, months from now, our doctor openly expresses his belief that our contributions may have been, if not a deal breaker, a serious contribution. Bless him for saying it, whether it is true or not.

Zen and the Art of Illness

I recall from my own illness experience years ago how I welcomed an afternoon car ride. It could be just back and forth to the bank. It could be just driving around and looking at the autumn colors. Anything. It was a sign of hope to be looking out a window. To this day, I am grateful for a mom who intuitively knew it was part of the path to recovery.

You have on your velcro slippers. They are spiffy enough no one will notice that you aren't wearing regular shoes. Your large grey sweatshirt is easy to get over your now slender body. The front of it sags where your chest once was. The shuffle to the car is slow but with intention. You need a little assistance to get the seat belt snapped correctly. There is a deep breath as we gently smile at each other. We know we won't be long. We have a silent understanding that doesn't need words. Getting out is important. And we are doing that.

It seems like months before you have the energy to do anything except sleep. I know it isn't. Sleep is actually difficult on some of the drugs. The days you take prednisone are the hardest. Exhausted but not sleeping is a version of torment. Dozing is the best you can do. As you graduate to television, there are many times I take the channel changer and mute the volume while you doze. There are days when I wish you would doze. During the period of time when your energy is sufficient to be sustained by television, I feel invaded by Law and Order, CSI, Law and Order, Missing, Law and Order, Law and Order, Law and Order. I don't have to be a psychologist to figure out you spent part of your life as a police officer. I wonder what people who are not former police officers watch when they are ill. I finally make a vow to myself. I will not personally watch more than one murder a day!

The months of chemotherapy are taking their toll. Each treatment is getting harder. Two more to go. The most noticeable unexpected side effect is that you are losing your voice. It isn't likely the chemo. It is the effort it takes to speak. You are assured, if it is the chemo, your voice will return. It makes for very quiet days. We are beginning to count the days.

One more chemotherapy to go. I sense the doubt in your eyes. Doubt coupled with determination. Can you do the whole treatment protocol? Late one evening after the last injection of the day, you smile that gentle smile that is your signature and add in your whispered voice, "All I have to do is show up tomorrow. If I can do that enough times, this will pass." A tear finds its way to the edge of my eye, and we both smile. I tuck you in. You never forget to say, "Thanks honey."

I accept that I have begun to run a split screen of my future, one with you, one without you. I need to know that I have the courage and the strength I need if fate is unkind.

In limbo, but home

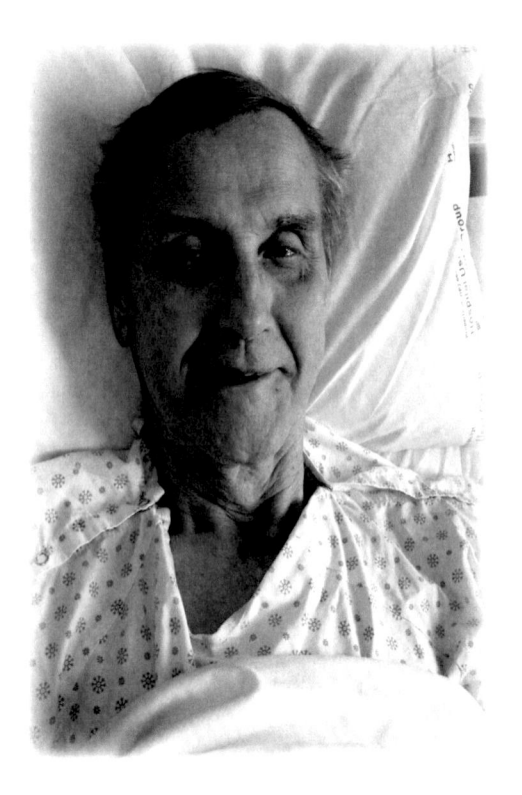

Zen and the Art of Illness

Your eyes are never without hope but they are consistently without energy. When you look at me, the gentleness of your nature quiets me. The going is getting tougher. How much can you take? Neither of us knows. We understand vulnerability in a new way. Today is what we have, and today we will touch each other gently. There have been no harsh words in more than thirty years. Today will not be the first.

I find myself reading. Reading. Reading. I am not wanting to escape. Rather, I am in search of inspiration. Not in a compulsive manner. A phrase of wisdom here. A statement of inspiration there. Thich Naht Hanh is calming. His writings remind me that my appointment with life is in the present moment. I remind myself "one day is a lot". There is time to be gentle, time to be together in a deep way, without words. I am wasting precious time if I spend it in resentment or regret. My moments of regret are acknowledged but are not privileged over gratitude. Denying a dark valley doesn't help me find a way out of it. I learned before this particular challenge that regret and fear are thieves of the moment.

Moments of fear, regret, and resentment are poor substitutes for moments of love.

Zen and the Art of Illness

The words of Thomas Merton, the Trappist monk, "our real journey in life is interior", remind me that I am creating my path by walking it. Resentment, fear, blame, discouragement are all intersections at which I must choose a direction. What is my interior destination? If I want peace, if I want courage, if I want patience, I have choices to make.

In limbo, but home

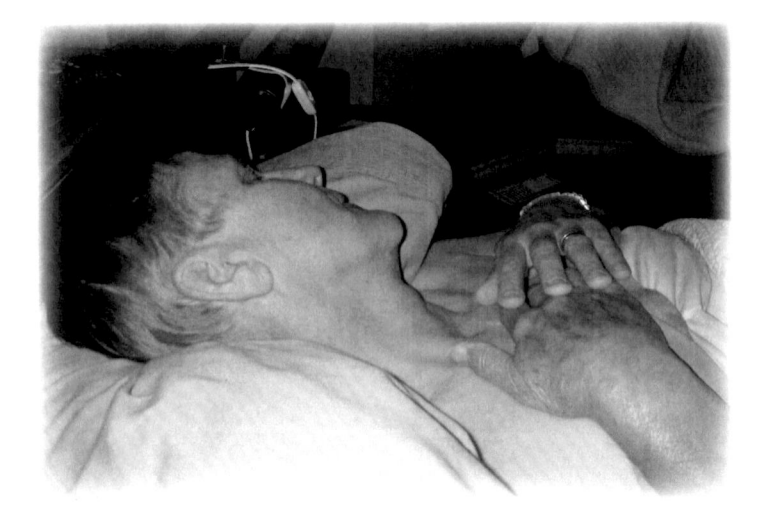

Zen and the Art of Illness

I am standing at the foot of your bed. You are resting peacefully. It is so good to see you resting peacefully. For that moment, I am hoping, simply hoping. On the day of your diagnosis, I heard myself whisper subvocally, "Please, let us have the summer." We have stolen time for many years. Or, perhaps been given it. Perhaps we will again be given more time. I am hoping for more than the summer. Not greed. Just hope. I am literally biting my upper lip so that the tears will stay inside. Not out of shame, or fear, or stoicism. Perhaps, at some point, somehow the tears will transform or inform. When they are ready, the tears will flow freely. But this is not the moment.

I have four university degrees. Surely I can figure out at least some of the basic computer problems I get myself into. It has been so easy to call "Al...len..." whenever I hit a glitch. Usually the solution is simple, and you smile as you lean over, hit a key or two, and my text returns. You never chastise me for not having mastered elementary procedures. Requesting a rescue these days is not an option. Somehow, I find the patience. I am gentle with myself as I explore solutions. But I miss your smile, your teasing eyes, and your technical competencies.

Zen and the Art of Illness

We knew the journey would not be easy. It was, however, the only path open to a cure, and it came without a guarantee. In the hospital, there is a kidney shaped plastic container for your emesis (vomit). At home, the empty large red coffee container is your constant companion. The anti-emetic (anti-nausea) medication is profoundly better than it was years ago. It isn't foolproof though. One morning the designated container is somewhere, somewhere other than where it needs to be. And there is no time. The garbage container suffices. You look up. The wet tears that accompany throwing up are more than from the retching. They are asking if this is going to be worth it. The tears in my eyes are asking the same question.

I kept the e-mails. All of them. For months. Evidence that people cared. I wonder if they know how important their well wishes and inquiries were. I wonder if I thanked them. More about that period of time than I would like to admit is a blur. At times, I forgot what information I shared with whom. Being more computer savvy would have been an asset. I don't know how to set up a group e-mail address list.

Zen and the Art of Illness

How many ways can I answer the question, "How is Allen?" It is months before you have the energy for even a brief telephone conversation. I am grateful for the inquiries. There are fewer and fewer over the months. People go back to their lives. I also notice my replies get shorter and shorter. I do my best to report small steps in the direction of health. I do my best to ask about their world.

I never knew what to reply to the e-mails that offered unsolicited prayer. I know what I would like to have said to the one or two who implied, and not so subtly, that our secular perspective on life was a contributing factor in the illness. I didn't share those tainted well wishes with you. Somehow there was a qualitative difference between the tone of those offerings and the quiet gifts of Dr. Cherry and Kuya. Despite the difference in their traditions, the message of compassion was not corrupted with implied deficits in us.

I am pleased that we have not been flooded by unsolicited advice. Perhaps my professional history inhibits people from offering what they might feel freer suggesting to family members or friends. It takes energy to graciously explain that what is being suggested is something we have been doing for years, or that we have absolutely no interest in trying the well intentioned offering. The issue is not really the advice. It is the style in which it is offered. It feels easy to detect in peoples' tone those who have a vested interest in us accepting their recommendations.

What do I say to the person who says, "Ronna, you have no life?" To the well intended who say, "You can't keep this up forever." But today, I can. I am not blind to my own needs. I know I cannot "do this" forever. At some point, I will have to take my life off hold. Right now, this is my life. Right now, this is my choice. It is not a choice for martyrdom. It is not a choice without thought. It is a willingness to be here. A willingness to be significant to only one person. For the moment, it is enough. If or when it is no longer enough, I will have to find a new way to navigate the ocean of illness, if we have not come to the shore.

Zen and the Art of Illness

There are times when I feel very alone. It is like living in an extended near-silent retreat. It isn't a feeling of loneliness. It is a sense of being "apart from". Of being completely out of the mainstream. It is hard to remember someone is selling carpet at the Bay, and people are sitting in meetings deciding things, that there are line-ups at fast food chains, and married couples are arguing about what tomorrow will bring.

Most of the time, I understand that people are choosing to be respectful by their absence, intending to protect my privacy during a difficult time.

At other times, I miss normalcy.

I wonder, "Do the kids know how ill he really is?" At one level, I know they have their own lives and challenges, and distance separates us. At another level, I long for them to call you more often. I long for them to know this special man who might go out of their lives. Mostly, I understand the bond is strong between all of us. On the days when I am sleep deprived, I long for them to magically appear. To be there at the very practical level. To prepare a cup of tea. To move a fallen tree. To have the car fueled. In those moments, it feels hard to be "growed up" so much of the time. I smile, and I make my own tea.

Zen and the Art of Illness

The mundane can be soothing. The garden is weeded. The ironing is done. The mirrors are polished. The vehicles are serviced. The bills are paid. The house is tidier and cleaner than usual. The bathroom is immaculate. There is no chance for a germ to attack your compromised immune system. If I can't control death, I can keep a clean house!

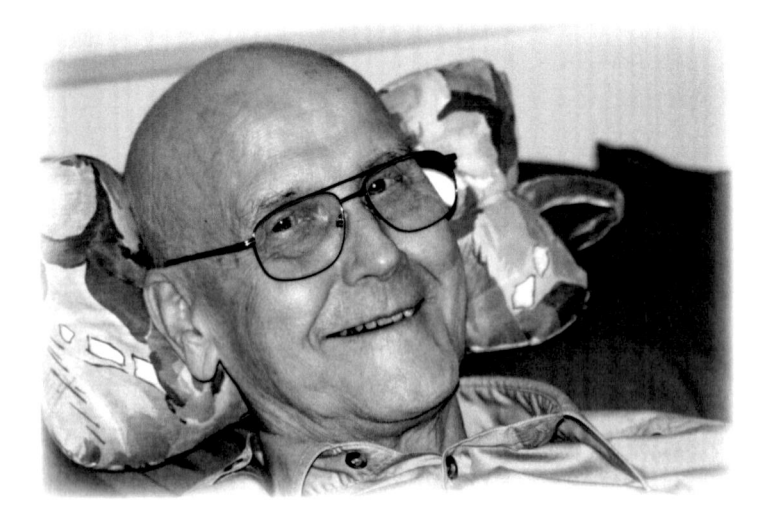

Zen and the Art of Illness

We never talked about the hair thing. It grew thinner. Then patchy. One day you announced, in a matter of fact way, "It's time". Ten minutes later, I am an amateur barber married to a bald man.

There are lots of comments. All positive. Suggestions that you are trendy, current with the many young men who choose shaven heads these days. I never, for even a moment, prefer you bald. There is something about looking at the person you have loved for three decades and straining to understand that he is the same man, just 45 pounds lighter with no hair.

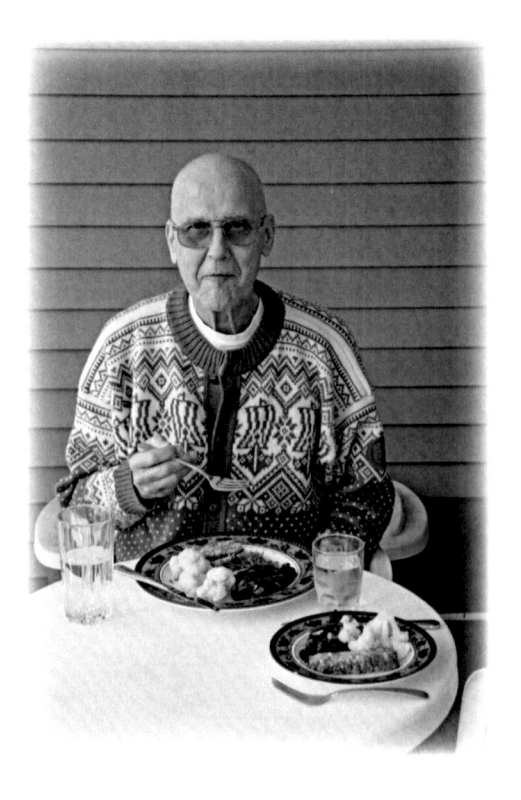

Zen and the Art of Illness

I know that I know you. Yet, there is something disconcerting about having lunch with someone who doesn't look like my husband. You don't look like the man with whom I have spent over thirty years. The eyes and the smile though, confirm it is you. But the hug is different. And the walk is different. I have to deliberately change channels to remember the you that I know. Without changing channels, I relate like a caregiver rather than a wife. I serve you a full plate knowing you will only nibble. It reminds me of the you that you were.

The cancer hospital is a research hospital. It came as no surprise that a research nurse entered our cubical in one of the later visits to inform us of a possible research protocol for which you might qualify. It would extend the chemo sessions a couple of months. We listened through the complicated preamble. You answered her questions. She was unsure if you would qualify with your heart history. She would let us know on the next visit. Neither of us were disappointed that you didn't qualify. If you had, I am not sure you would have agreed.

At some level we both knew, this chemotherapy was all that you could take.

Zen and the Art of Illness

As we near the hospital on the day of your last chemotherapy, there is something different. Not the usual slight, or not so slight, signs of anxiety. I can't quite put my finger on it as we turn down University Avenue. I ask, "Are you okay?" With a strength that doesn't seem possible given your fatigue, you reply, "I am getting ready. I am going to walk into that hospital and walk out. I want Dr. Reiman to see what he has created." There is no smile. No hint of anything except what I used to think of as your policeman deportment. I like how it feels though.

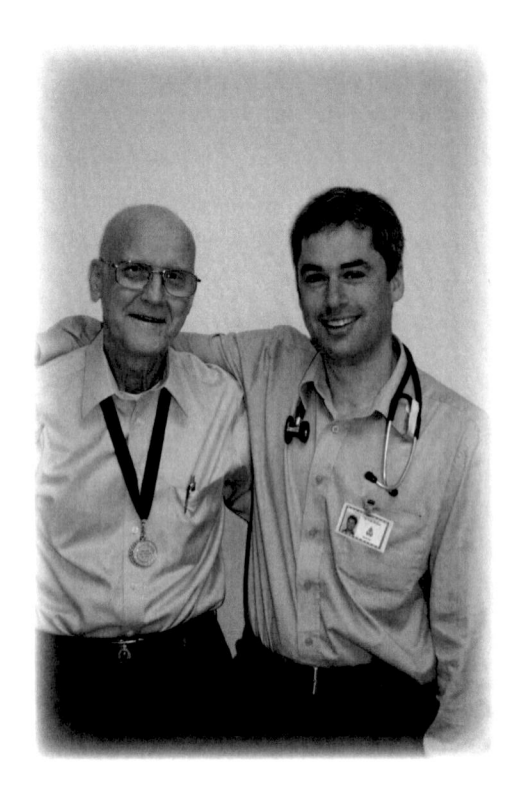

Zen and the Art of Illness

The day has finally come. Today, following your blood results, you will have your last chemotherapy. Dr. Reiman arrives smiling, extends his hand, and a warmth passes between all of us. He opens with "Mr. Eng, when I first met you, I set the bar pretty low. There is no reason now to lower it." He compliments us for our contribution to the process. I ask if we could have a photo. I am not sure what was more noticeable - your sense of relief or Dr. Reiman's brimming smile. Before I take the photo, I present you with an Olympic medal around your neck. On the back it reads "You are my miracle".

This morning we said our goodbyes to Dr. Reiman who is leaving soon for New Brunswick. You have had your final chemotherapy. You are at home tucked into the flannel sheets that seem to give you comfort. It is 6:40 p.m.. I promised to be at the poolside by 7:00 p.m. Now though, I stand at the base of the bed. My swimming gear is nearby. My cell phone is in my hand. I call Nicole. It is a call to Lethbridge. We love our new grand daughter-in-law. She is with her friend, her brother, and our granddaughter. Our grandsons are both working and will swim later. The call is short and simple. We are "good to go."

I bow, literally bow, to you and explain we are all about to do "an honor swim". Each of us will swim one kilometer in honor of your chemotherapy journey. You have done something difficult, and we want to show our appreciation by doing something that takes effort. I have been training for three months for this day. I reached my goal only four days before the honor swim. The swim is our way of recognizing the effort you have put in. I love that memory. No words. Just a bow and two people who love each other, smiling. And four kids, three hundred miles away honoring grandpa. Can life get any better?

RETURNING TO LIFE:
Finding normal again

The only Zen you can find
on the tops of mountains
is the Zen you bring up there.

Robert M. Pirsig

This is the first day in six months that we don't have to take your vital signs. It feels foreign to leave the rituals of vigilance behind. Can you really be okay enough that we don't have to check for abnormalities four times a day? We don't have to chart. We still have the "What if" directions that the hospital provided in the top drawer of your bedside table. "If this, then that." We remind ourselves how grateful we are that once the cancer hospital took you on, they were always there for us. We don't have to go through channels to address a fever or an unexpected symptom.

We are not free yet. You have though been granted a promotion. No more shots. The thermometer though will stay nearby for a couple of weeks. We will graduate towards normalcy.

Zen and the Art of Illness

Do I push or do I pamper? Finding the balance between inviting you to start to strengthen and respecting the deep fatigue these months have left you with is something we negotiate together. The road back will be long and we know we will need patience. Lots of patience. I feel the need to return to work, at least part time. Occasionally, I long to be pampered even for a hour. That time will come. I too have some recovering to do. I am weary from being on alert for months.

Life begins a series of firsts. Instead of first chemo, first injection, first follow up, we are entering a new series of firsts - first tea, first walk, first ice cream, first university class, first push-up.

Zen and the Art of Illness

For years, we have had tea once a week. Before the illness, it was Monday mornings. It is a time for aligning schedules, setting priorities, talking things through. Sometimes, there is time enough to exchange views on something one of us is reading. Our tea room is a retreat for us. We shut the world out. We don't answer the phone. It is an hour for just us. The first day we manage tea in the tea room is like a celebration. You last almost a half hour, and all we do is smile. There is no agenda. There is just the return of a treasured ritual.

Although our journey has required me to be a caregiver, sometimes on an hourly basis, I am aware that we have been partners, that we are partners, in this venture. We are companions on this pilgrimage. It is not solely me helping you. It is us doing the best we can to navigate this difficult landscape. You support me as I support you. Only once have you uttered a mildly harsh phrase, and it injured you more than me. It was easy to assure you that, in that moment, you were not the Allen you wanted to be. Even in that moment, we could be companions. One companion can be momentarily difficult. It doesn't cancel the depth of friendship or the thousand genuine thank yous over the difficult months.

Zen and the Art of Illness

Doug has left us with all six episodes of Star Wars. I join you on the reclining love seat and the whole day passes. Your stamina is such that you nap between episodes. I let go of expecting anything from myself except to be present. It is a satisfying day, just letting go of the need to "do". What a privilege to be able to do so. It is a difficult time in our lives. The timing, though, is such that we can do much of it together. I have stopped seeing clients to ensure that we can be together. So that we can do what friends do.

Finding normal again

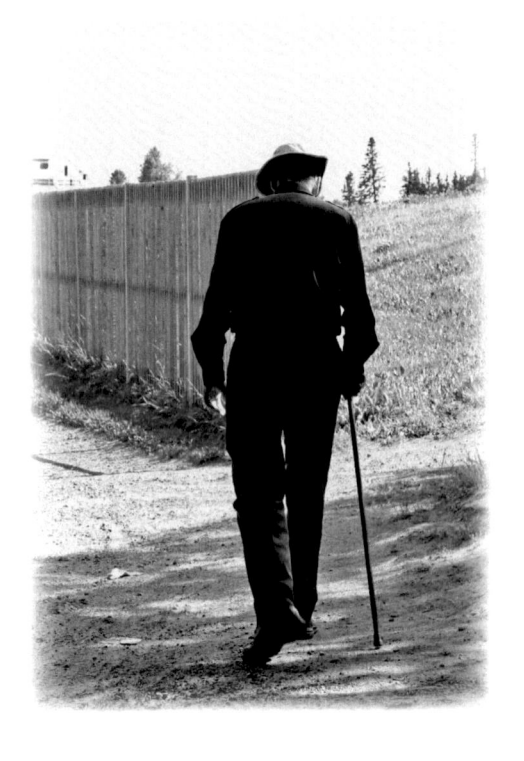

Zen and the Art of Illness

There is a strange solace in that you were diagnosed in winter, treated in the spring, and we have the summer for recovery. That first little walk beyond the front steps is like the entry onto a remembered stage. Yes, this is what we do, this is who we are. We are going for our morning walk. No matter that it is not far. Laughingly not far.

And getting back feels like having climbed Everest.

Being back is a triumph.

The teas with others begin. People begin to connect again. Mostly for tea. "We won't stay long. Just a cup of tea." It doesn't matter that it is often longer and that you often withdraw in your gracious way. Each tea is like a yard toward the goal posts of normal activity. Despite your smiles, the weariness shows at times. There is no doubt though, that people feel welcome, grateful at your efforts to be present for the visit. Grateful that their friend will survive.

Zen and the Art of Illness

For a while life seems like a series of teas. Thank goodness, I am friends with muffin making. The ritual of tea is an invitation to make room in life for conversation. To just be. It's not a meeting. There's no agenda. With luck the muffins are fresh, the jelly is home made, and the tea is steeped in a china pot. The fridge magnet is right again, "Where there is tea, there is hope."

Convinced your immune system is recovering, we're ready for a meal in public. The big adventure is tofu vegetable soup at the Wok and Roll, our favorite soup in our favorite restaurant. When you had a heart attack just days after we were married years ago, we agreed to "make memories". As the soup arrived, we smiled and almost simultaneously said, "Makin' memories". Just tofu vegetable soup and green tea. That's all it takes. And gratitude for being alive and having each other.

Zen and the Art of Illness

Our first long outing is a drive to Camrose, 40 kilometers away. We dawdled through the countryside, noticing the damage from the recent storm, the low levels of the creeks. Any one who thinks global warming is a conspiracy dreamed up by environmental extremists need only drive through the disappearing landscape. Lunch is at the Lefse House that serves authentic Scandinavian food. We are surprised to see the packed house in their new premises. Graciously a woman of my vintage sitting with an elderly woman motions that we are welcome to share their table. We learn it is Aunt Edith's 97th birthday lunch and a new friendship begins.

Dr. Goa helped keep the hope alive. There is a place in our heart for him that no one else will occupy. With each visit, he leaves the impression you will complete his course. There is something motivating in the positively offered expectation. His visits to our home in the ensuing weeks make me think, if this was a movie, his part might be played by Anthony Hopkins in the way Hopkins played C.S. Lewis. You would sit supported with a big pillow in the recliner in the living room. I would provide gluten-free goodies, since our guest was a newly diagnosed celiac. For the next approximately 45 minutes to an hour, I would remove myself. The philosophy talk would begin. I listened for the time when silence exceeded speech and would reappear. I know he has given you an extension on your paper. How do you thank someone for transcending the probable and attending to the possible?

Zen and the Art of Illness

It is inconceivable to me that you have completed the required term paper. Many times, I found you with a book tipped onto your chest while you slept. Somehow, book after book was inviting you back to normalcy. Somehow, the gears of thought were grinding from a halt back to active status. You got an A. You intend to return to university in the fall.

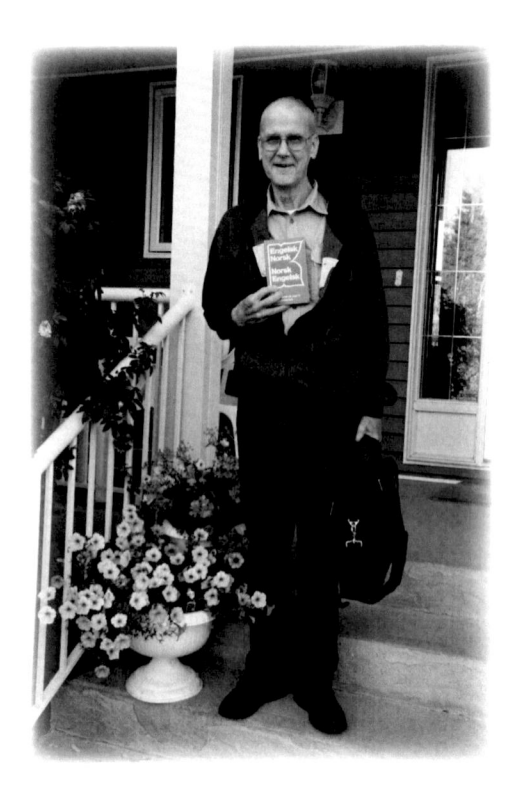

Zen and the Art of Illness

It is hard to imagine that you are actually going off to university again. Bald head. Cane in hand. A bit wobbly but proud. I keep my hope silent. I had hoped that you would hold back, and not demand so much of yourself. At some level, I understand. The sooner your life resembles the life that you lost, the more it will feel like it could be what it was.

Despite your weakness, your arm reaches out as the room darkens. I love the big windows in our bedroom. The moon is full, the treetops outlined against the sky. The kind of night when a late evening walk would be mystical. My first moments of sleep are snuggled into your shoulder. There is the illusion of being safe and for those moments, we are.

Zen and the Art of Illness

Looking up at you from my pillow, our eyes meet. Another milestone. You are up before me and are bringing me hot water and lemon, a ritual that has not happened for many months. Strange how little things feel like major benchmarks. We both smile. I offer "Thanks, hon." You offer, "You're welcome." In silence, we know another bridge had been crossed.

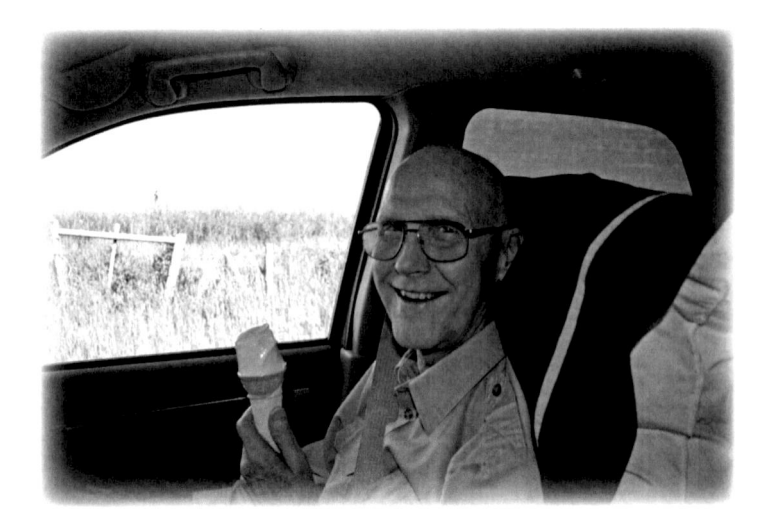

Zen and the Art of Illness

Ice cream is not vegan, but then,

our eating regime is not a religion.

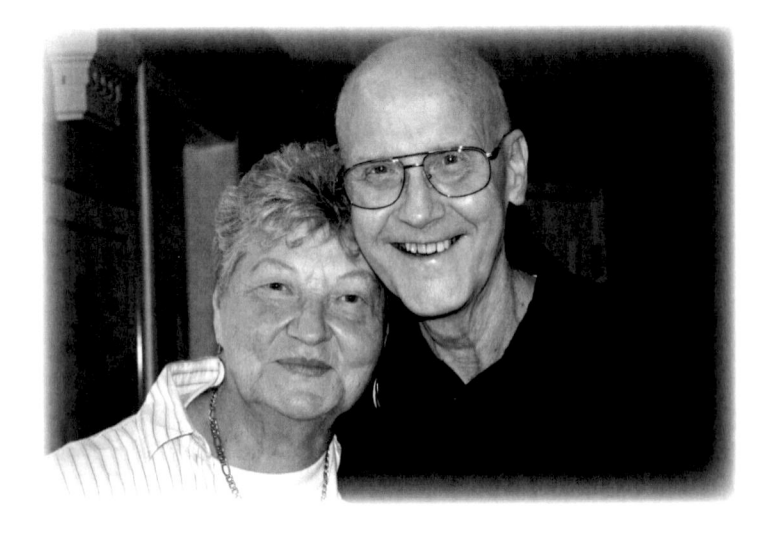

Zen and the Art of Illness

There is something to be said about old friends. Dad used to say, "It is one thing to make new friends. It is another to lose the friends you made the memories with." Gloria's visit meant so much to you. Childhood friends never lose that special place in our hearts. And age makes speaking the truth so much easier.

There is daily evidence of hope. You are puttering in your office, making the occasional phone call, asking about people, walking about the garden. One day, you sharpen the knives. I know my Allen is coming back. My Allen loves sharp knives. And you have enough energy for short conversations.

Zen and the Art of Illness

When I asked if you ever lost hope, your reply was a simple "No". When I asked if you had been afraid at any time, I was surprised at your definitive "Yes!". You added that you were concerned because you had not taught me our finance program. You had failed to adequately prepare me to do the accounts! That was it. Not fear about death. Not conscious fear about recurrence. Not concern that you might never drive again. There are advantages to being a practical kinda' guy.

Finding normal again

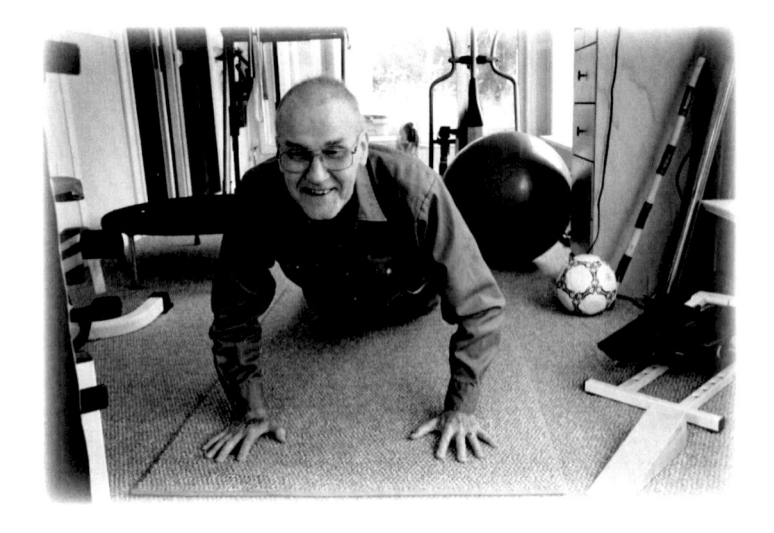

Zen and the Art of Illness

"Ronna, can you bring your camera?"

"Sure. Where are you?"

"I am in the fitness room."

I enter the fitness room that we love, the fitness room that you and Nels built for me when I was recovering from a motor vehicle accident that required months of physiotherapy. With windows on three sides, the light streams in.

"I thought you might want a picture of this. I am going to try to do a push up."

Prostrate on the Berber rug, you look up for a moment while I capture your first push up. Rather, your first effort at a push up. It warms my heart to see your intent. We both laugh.

Finding normal again

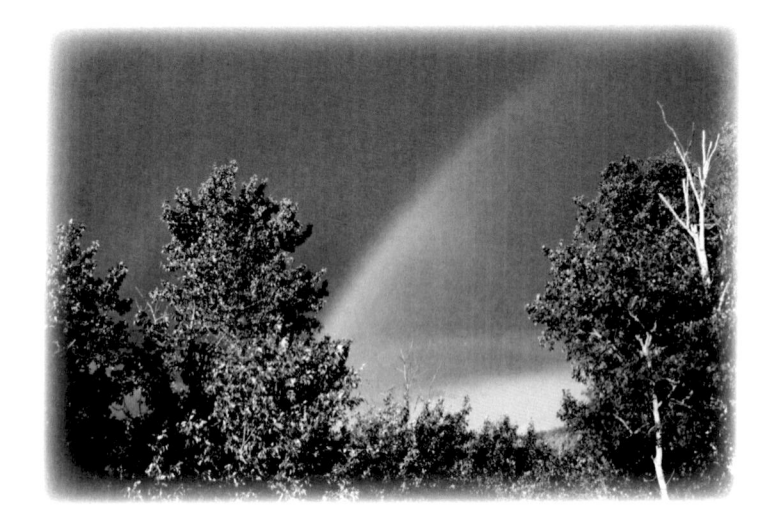

Zen and the Art of Illness

There is something wonderful about watching a summer storm. Something metaphorical. The horizon darkens. There is often the quiet before the storm, the perfect stillness of apprehension. The foreshadowing leaves no doubt as the winds begin. The trees start to sway. There is the lighting that happens only as storms approach. The lightning and thunder are like an unpredictable concert that plays itself out before the downpour begins. Then, the silence again. The postcard stillness. The freshness. The rare lighting that photographers wait hours for. Then, the mystery of a rainbow.

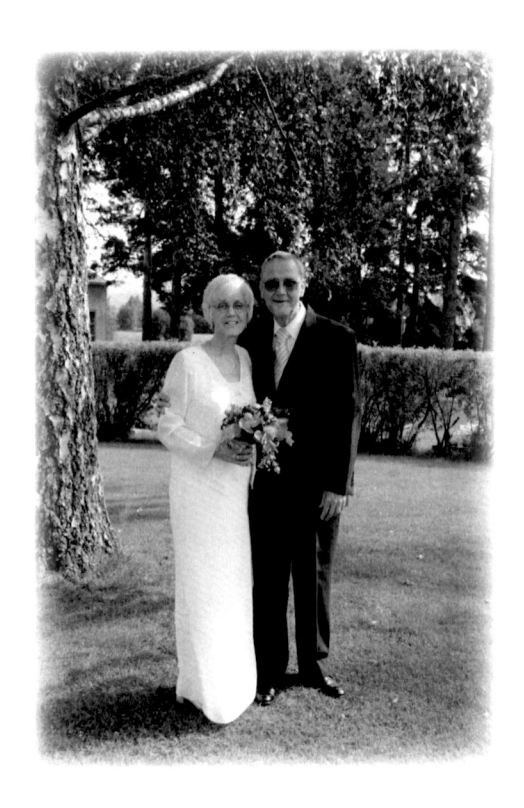

Zen and the Art of Illness

It's three years now. Three years since we took each day as it came. Three years since we walked the walk that no one chooses voluntarily. This year we journeyed to Sweden to the village of Farila where we celebrated our 30th anniversary by renewing our vows in the cathedral in which your ancestors have been married for the last four centuries. Now, on this anniversary of one hundred years since your family left for the new world, we returned to say to each other the vows we took so naively years ago. In the interim, we have learned not only to navigate the storms, but to dance in the rain. The love and the commitment are deeper for having had challenges on the journey.

Epilogue

After enlightenment, comes the laundry.

> Zen proverb

Cherry trees will blossom every year;
But I'll disappear for good,
One of these days.

> Philip Whalen

Epilogue 2

Allen passed away September 8, 2013 after yet another pilgrimage with yet another primary cancer. His legacy is a deep and quiet courage that he shared with all of those who loved him.

About the Author

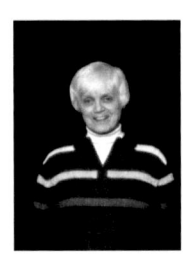

Ronna Fay Jevne

Ronna Jevne is a professor emeritus of the University of Alberta. Her career has spanned decades as a teacher, psychologist, professor, inspirational speaker, and the author of more than a dozen books.

Ronna was a founding member of the Canadian Association of Psychosocial Oncology, and of the Hope Foundation of Alberta (now Hope Studies Central), at the University of Alberta.

She shares her love of writing, particularly reflective writing, with students, patients, health care professionals, high needs adolescents, inmates, correctional officers, and many others who enjoy the benefits of writing to enhance well-being.

Ronna lives in a quiet rural setting with her husband, Hal and their red heeler, Spirit.

Ronna and Hal share their commitment to writing through the Prairie Wind Writing Centre.

prairiewindwritingcentre.ca